DEDICATION

This book is dedicated to my Patty – daddy's little girl. I will be here always and I promise to hold your hand through your first heartache until you find that perfect man. That's how much I love you, baby girl.

TABLE OF CONTENTS

How to Be Healthier One Bite at a Time

Tips on How to Get the Perfect Weight without Resorting to Diet Plan Fads

By: Kevin Jones

9781635014891

PUBLISHERS NOTES

Disclaimer – Speedy Publishing LLC

This publication is intended to provide helpful and informative material. It is not intended to diagnose, treat, cure, or prevent any health problem or condition, nor is intended to replace the advice of a physician. No action should be taken solely on the contents of this book. Always consult your physician or qualified health-care professional on any matters regarding your health and before adopting any suggestions in this book or drawing inferences from it.

The author and publisher specifically disclaim all responsibility for any liability, loss or risk, personal or otherwise, which is incurred as a consequence, directly or indirectly, from the use or application of any contents of this book.

Any and all product names referenced within this book are the trademarks of their respective owners. None of these owners have sponsored, authorized, endorsed, or approved this book.

Always read all information provided by the manufacturers' product labels before using their products. The author and publisher are not responsible for claims made by manufacturers.

This book was originally printed before 2014. This is an adapted reprint by Speedy Publishing LLC with newly updated content designed to help readers with much more accurate and timely information and data.

Speedy Publishing LLC

40 E Main Street, Newark, Delaware, 19711

Contact Us: 1-888-248-4521

Website: http://www.speedypublishing.co

REPRINTED Paperback Edition: 9781635014891:

Manufactured in the United States of America

Chapter 1- Why Is It Important to Eat Healthy?

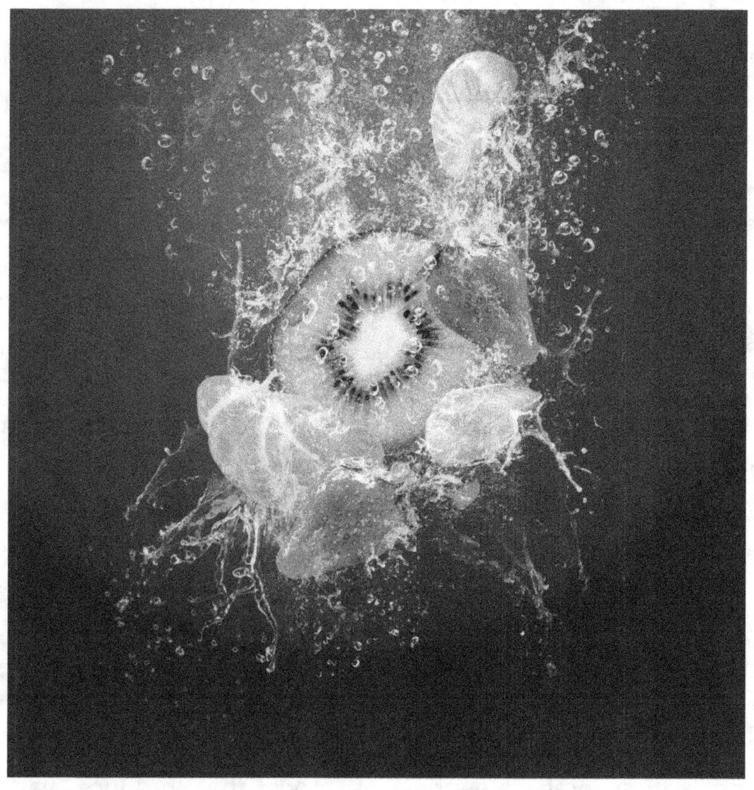

Energy is needed for the various functions like maintenance of growth, daily activities, exercise and many other movements or functions that are often taken for granted. These are shared between the two energy systems.

In today's world, seldom do any health and fitness plans work. What's the reason for their alarming rate of failure?

The world is a lot less healthful than it was two decades ago. Much this is attributed to the altered food habits of individuals.

The primary and first to be used energy system is the aerobic system. This system uses oxygen for the function of the muscles and does demand quite a lot from the general body system.

This demand usually increases the rate and depth of breathing and blood supply mainly because of the corresponding increase of the heart rate.

When the body requires more energy which cannot be met due to the elevated need for more oxygen then the body system automatically switched to the anaerobic energy system. This system is able to produce energy without the need to use oxygen.

All this energy is generated through the suitable or correct consumption of foods. The foods consumed dictate the types of energy levels each individual is capable of producing.

Muscle fatigue usually occurs when all the energy sources are exhausted which can be attributed to a variety of reasons; the most compelling one depends very much on the types of foods consumed.

There are several categories of foods that produce various beneficial elements for the human body system and noting the ones that create or enhance the energy generating sources is definitely useful to know. Therefore this knowledge should help the individual choose the right types of foods.

The aerobic system works by breaking down the carbohydrates, fatty acids and amino acids in the foods consumed while the anaerobic system releases energy from the foods stored in the body, usually during intense activity bouts.

If we hear about the failure of diets or gym plans all around us, commonly it isn't their fault. Commonly it is the fault of the individuals who started with much commotion about going through these plans, telling all their acquaintances and co-workers about it, and then didn't abide by those programs.

The individuals who abandon the exercise or diet halfway do not see the advantages, naturally, and everybody blames the plan.

What the world needs nowadays isn't a fresh health or fitness program or a diet, but it requires motivation. It needs the correct sort of mind-set to follow through with whatever plan they have chosen to the very end.

If they can do that, most of the health issues that are related to life-style situations will get to be outmoded. And we don't have to visit the corners of the earth to discover this motivation. The motivation lies right here, inside us; we simply need to search it out and utilize it.

One generation ago, individuals wouldn't dream of picking up whatever junk food they could get in order to feed their faces. Nowadays, we do that so very casually. "I'm hungry" commonly means "I want a burger or a hot dog, likely with chips on the side and some cola." And, "I am on a diet" means "I am on a chemically ridden pill which will defeat my hunger and deprive my body of vitamins." It's genuinely no wonder that we are facing so many health issues today.

Our health is an indicator of what we consume. The sorry condition that we're living in isn't an individual problem; it's a global issue. The world as a whole is eating incorrectly. Six in every ten individuals in the US is overweight, and the number is going to be eight in every ten individuals by the time we hit 2015.

Are we truly thinking about this? We aren't. Even as you're studying this eBook, you likely have a packet of chips on the side. Do you know that what you spent on that package, which is filling your stomach with some of the most toxic chemicals known to humanity, could instead have fed an emaciated youngster in Ruanda?

But it's not simply about being philanthropic. It's about us too. Yes, we have to be selfish. With such appalling health figures, aren't we heading for doom? We're definitely not eating right. Whatever excess baggage that brings - obesity and the assorted ill health in its wake - we have to be prepared for it.

The Pros of Eating Healthy

There are several reasons and benefits of healthy eating and thus you should remove time to prepare healthy food and chalk out a diet for a healthy living. Here are the benefits of healthy eating:

• Apart from feeling and looking good, your body will be high on energy, and fresh. With healthy eating, you enjoy doing everything, and live a full life. Healthy eating leads to a healthier you and you find little or no reason to visit a doctor. You can spend time in more activities to keep fit.

• As a healthy diet keeps the immune system stronger, and health problems are kept far away. A healthy immune system will take care that you stay fit and if sick to recover fast.

• Healthy diets help you stay in shape. A well-planned and healthy food helps to maintain your weight and you save yourself from the worry of losing or gaining weight.

- Your brain gets alert and sharp, which helps you to perform well in all your activities. A research has proved that a healthy diet helps your mind to think well even in the old age. You must have seen people fit and fine even in late 80's and all this is the result of proper food intake.

- A wholesome diet gives you all the essential minerals and nutrients that fulfill all the needs of your body.

- A healthy diet has proved to keep humans in a happy mood. Hence, you enjoy every moment of life and stay calm in every situation.

- Your skin is the face of your body. You know what the secret for a glowing skin is? It is healthy food. This not only makes you look great, but you feel strengthened from within.

- A good diet is very important for growing kids. Children are very active, burn lot of calories, and thus require all the required proteins, carbs, fats, and nutrients to stay fit and not affect their growth in any way.

Many people who have ignored bad eating habits have regretted in the older years. Healthy food keeps away many diseases and ill effects and you live a life that is free of tension and problems. Apart from enjoying life, you develop positive feelings. Therefore, healthy food keeps both mind and body fit for life long. Thus, it is never too late to begin to eat healthy food and so live a healthy life. You will never run into bad effects because of good eating habits. So it is always better to eat well and stay in good shape. You can keep obesity and other harmful health problems far away from you.

Eating and Surviving

Survival of the fittest is the one single principle that rules the animal world. This rule does not govern humanity, however, and as a result, man has relegated health to the bottom of his priority list. It is only when nature provides a shocking reminder of neglect through a stroke or a heart attack that most people realize that they should have followed a healthy routine.

There are a few simple steps to follow to be in good health. Regular exercise and intake of the right foods to keep your body fit, and develop a strong immune system to fight the onslaught of various diseases. Eat the correct proportion of fats, proteins and carbohydrates to provide the vitamins, minerals and other elements needed by the body to survive, and flourish.

Carbohydrates rich foods have a combination of fiber, sugar and starch, and thus supply the body with glucose that provides the energy to complete physical tasks. Proteins too are vital in providing energy to the body, but you need to watch out for foods that have healthy and unhealthy levels of fat along with protein. The right combination of fresh vegetables, fruits, and dairy and meat products can fulfil your body's needs. This means that you can perform all the physical tasks while your brain too remains healthy and active.

A fit body and mind not only ensures a long and healthy life, but also keeps all major and minor diseases at bay. A healthy mind and body can delay any age related disease, such as Alzheimer's or osteoporosis thus improving the quality of life. Promote healthy eating habits among your loved ones and your children. The right foods help you increase your efficiency while exercising and during work. A healthy mind keeps stress at bay, and this result in a general sense of well-being, and contentment.

On the other hand, eating unhealthy food over a long period can lead to fat accumulating in various parts of your body including your arteries. While body fat is easily visible, fat accumulating inside your body is not visible and unfortunately is irreversible. Thus, you might have to go in for a heart bypass operation to replace clogged arteries, if you ignore your health for a long time. The key is to embark on healthy eating habits from childhood itself. For girls and women too, healthy eating habits can result in flawless skin and a fit body. The right combination of a heavy breakfast, medium lunch, and a light dinner can help the body to digest in a more efficient way.

As the old saying goes, 'prevention is better than cure' and by embarking on a mission to eat healthy foods, you can ensure that you live a long and healthy life. A healthy diet enables you to perform all physical and mental functions, while ensuring that you live a better quality of life, free from any ailments.

CHAPTER 2- HOW TO BECOME A HEALTHY EATER

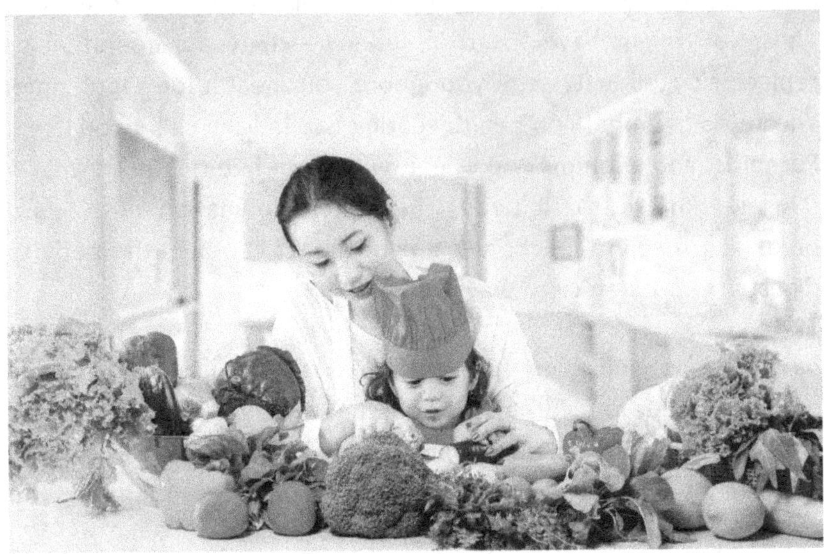

Being a healthy eater requires you to become both educated and smart about what healthy eating actually is. Being food smart isn't about learning to calculate grams of fat, and it isn't about studying labels and counting calories. Healthy eating is all about balanced and moderate eating, consisting of healthy meals at least three times per day.

Healthy eaters eat many different types of foods, not limiting themselves to one specific food type or food group. Eating healthy requires quite a bit of leeway. You might eat too much or not enough consume foods that are sometimes more or less nutritious. However, you should always fuel your body and your brain regularly with enough food to keep both your mind and body strong and alert.

A healthy eater is a good problem solver. Healthy eaters have learned to take care of themselves and their eating with sound judgment and making wise decisions. Healthy eaters are always aware of what they eat, and know the effect that it will have on their bodies. When someone is unable to take control of their eating, they are also likely to get out of control with other aspects of life as well. They could end up spending too much, talking too much, and even going to bed later and later.

You should always remember that restricting food in any way is always a bad thing. Healthy eating is a way of life, something that you can do to enhance your body or your lifestyle. If you've thought about making your life better, healthy eating is just the place to start. You'll make life easier for yourself, those around you, and even your family.

Busting Myths on Eating

1. Working out on an empty stomach.

If you hear a rumbling noise in your stomach, the rumbling is trying to tell you something. If you don't listen to your stomach, you are forcing your body to run without any fuel. Before you exercise or do any physical activity, always eat a light snack such as an apple.

2. Relying on energy bars and drinks.

Although they are fine every once in a while, they don't deliver the antioxidants you need to prevent cancer. Fruits and vegetables are your best bets, as they are loaded in vitamins, minerals, fluid, and fiber.

3. Skipping breakfast.

Skipping breakfast is never a good idea, as breakfast starts the day. Your body needs fuel as soon as possible, and without it, you'll be hungry throughout the day.

4. Low carb diets.

Your body needs carbohydrates for your muscles and the storing of energy.

5. Eating what you want.

Eating healthy and exercising doesn't give you an all access pass to eat anything you want. Everyone needs the same nutrients whether they exercise or not, as well as fruits and vegetables.

6. Not enough calories.

Although losing weight involves calories, losing it too quickly is never safe. What you should do, is aim for 1 - 2 pounds a week. Always make sure that you are getting enough calories to keep your body operating smoothly. If you start dropping weight too fast, eat a bit more food.

7. Skip soda and alcohol.

Water, milk, and juice are the best to drink for active people. You should drink often, and not require on thirst to be an indicator. By the time you get thirsty, your body is already running a bit too low.

Changing how you eat is always a great step towards healthy eating and it will affect how your body performs. The healthier you eat, the better you'll feel. No matter how old you may be, healthy eating is something you should strive for. Once you give it a chance, you'll see in no time at all just how much it can change your life - for the better.

It's The Way You Think about Food

We have strayed horribly with our eating habits thus far. Unless we take stock of the state of affairs and take matters in our own hands, matters are not going to get better.

The number 1 thing is awareness. We have to learn what foods are correct for us and what are not. We have to go back to training and comprehend what the nutrients are that your body truly wants and in what amount.

Then we have to build a dietary regimen for ourselves and our loved ones so that we eat healthier. We have to cut down on all the foods that are adverse - the sugars, the fats, the carbohydrates, we don't truly want them - and incorporate foods that may boost our health.

This does sound too preachy, I understand. But that's the only reprieve we have got. If we continue munching on Oreos, we're never going to get better.

But there's hope. Hope lies in the fact that there are a lot of foods out there that are simply as tasty as those awful junk foods but we don't yet know about them.

These are the foods that we don't know about yet, we likely don't care for them or as we don't know how to fix them, but a healthy cookbook may help you in understanding assorted interesting ways to healthy cooking.

Even with the same sort of diet you eat, you are able to conjure up some really delicious healthy dishes. Yes, it's all very much possible. You are able to modify your eating habits to a big extent, while at the same time attending to your palate.

The fact is that the weight loss industry is responsible in a really significant way towards this downfall of the developed human race. They have to keep selling their Atkinses and Jenny Craigs and Zones and Medifasts and for that reason the media never tells you how we may in reality take things in your own hands.

They show us glitzy before-after pictures of a person with a foot-long sub and then the same guy with 6 pack abs and tell us that the diet made that possible.

However the fact is if we were to get our head together, we may very easily do that too, without having to spend 1000s of dollars on those diets. And what do we have to do?

2 general things:-

Control what we consume.

Indulge in physical exertion.

Now, is that too much to accomplish? Don't we owe that to our body that has served us so well all these years? Don't we owe that to ourselves and our loved ones?

CHAPTER 3- CHOOSE THE HEALTHIER OPTIONS

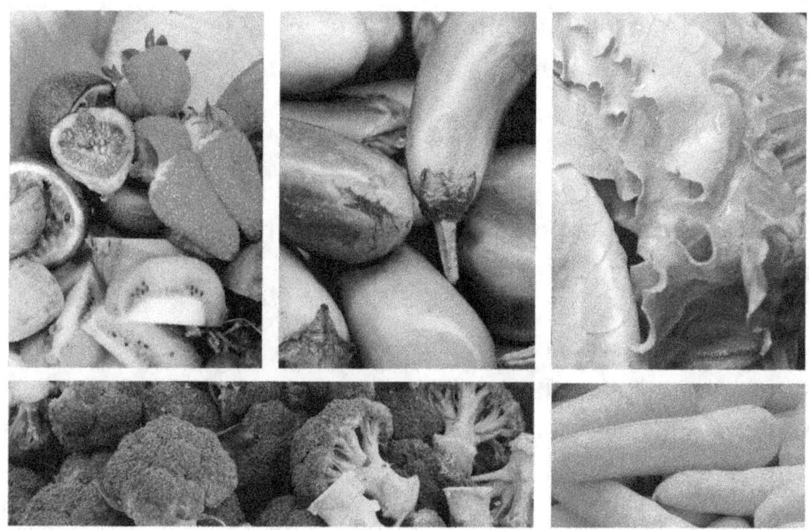

Vegetables, fruits, and grains are normally low in fat and have no cholesterol. Most are great sources of dietary fiber, complex carbs, and vitamins. The American Heart Association recommends that you eat foods that are high in complex carbs and fiber.

Below are some tips for making healthy food choices.

Coconut is high in saturated fat, while olives are high in mono unsaturated fats and calories. You should use these items sparingly to avoid getting too many calories from fat.

When vegetable grains are cooked, saturated fat or cholesterol is often added. For example, egg yolks may be added to bread or even pasta.

Processed, canned, or preserved vegetables may also contain added sodium. With some people, too much sodium, salt, may lead to high blood pressure. There are some food companies that are actually canning vegetables with less salt. You can look for these in the market area or choose fresh and even frozen vegetables.

Nuts and seeds tend to be high in calories and fat, although a majority of the fat is polyunsaturated or mono unsaturated. There are some varieties, macadamia nuts for example, that are also high in saturated fat.

Foods that are high in soluble fiber are a great choice as well. Examples include oat bran, oatmeal, beans, peas, rice bran, barley, and even apple pulp.

Whenever you are looking for healthy food choices, always make sure you read the nutrition label or information about the food. You can then determine what the food contains and how healthy it truly is for your body. By taking your time and making your healthy food choices wisely, you'll have a lifetime to enjoy the foods that will take care of you.

About Honey and Whole Grains

Over the years honey has been proven to the one sustaining power behind the energy circle. Benefiting the human body in various areas it is foremost still unrivaled in its energy producing entity. Honey is nature's most natural energy booster. It also acts as an effective immunity system builder while providing the natural remedy to a host of varied ailments too.

Energy is very important to the smooth flowing natural of a daily life cycle of any human being. Therefore finding energy sources that are both consistent and healthy are important to keeping fit and happy.

The natural benefits of honey has been widely acknowledged and accepted. Besides its great taste, honey is also a natural source of carbohydrate, which is an energy maker for boosting performance, endurance and reducing levels of muscle fatigue.

This is especially useful for athletes. The sugar content in the honey helps to play a role in preventing fatigue during exercise sessions and also during training sessions for sports enthusiast. These sugar make ups are divided into glucose and fructose and functions in different but complimenting ways.

The glucose content in the honey is generally absorbed at a faster rate and gives off an immediate energy boost while the fructose works at a slower pace for a more sustainable and prolonged energy use. When it comes to addressing blood sugar levels in the body system, honey has been known to help keep the levels fairly constant.

As honey is a pleasant food product and it's natural in its form, consuming it is not a very difficult exercise. People of all ages are generally quite willing to consume honey in any of its accompanying forms. It's even popular with children.

The energy produced from consuming a small amount of honey daily helps children cope with the physical strains of daily school activities and sports commitments. For the adults too consuming a daily small dose of honey can go a long way in keeping the energy levels at its best during a demanding day at work.

Making sandwiches with honey accompanied with other fillings is one way of creating a pleasant snack. Applying honey on a freshly toasted slice of bread is also a welcome breakfast alternative. Adding honey to drinks instead of using sugar is definitely encouraged.

How To Be Healthier One Bite At A Time

Most people today want a quick fix for their energy boosting needs and this usually comes in the unhealthy forms of sports drinks, coffee and refined carbohydrates like sugar and while bread.

Though these produce the desired heightened energy levels, it should be noted that this energy is fairly short lived and the tiredness that follows is usually more acutely felt. Therefore opting to consume some form of whole grains is not only a better alternative but is also much healthier.

Whole grains provide the energy that comes in a more complex form which breaks down over a longer period of time. This then creates the platform for sustaining the energy levels for longer periods.

Because of its more complex make up the whole grains come with an array of beneficial elements like minerals, vitamins, phytonutrients and fiber which are also rich in fiber.

Adding the whole grain ingredients is any dish more often than not completes the flavor or enhances it altogether. Whole grains can the various forms such as wheat, oat, barley, maize, brown rice, faro, spelt, emmer, einkorn, rye, millet, buckwheat, and many more.

These can then be made into various other products like whole wheat flour, whole wheat bread, whole wheat pasta, rolled oats, triticale flour, popcorn and teff flour.

The benefits of consuming whole grains consistently can help decrease the risk of heart disease, lower cholesterol levels protect against many types of cancer and assist in weight management. Whole grains should not be confused with its lesser and more refined "cousin". Though refined grains have some benefits it is always better to opt for the whole grain alternatives.

About Nuts and Lean Meat

Nuts are an important source of nutrients for both human and animal consumption. Being rich in a whole host of necessary nutrients it can be eaten in its raw form, cooked or as an additive to already preexisting dishes. Thought nuts are defined as a hard shelled fruit, there are many other foods that are included in the nut family.

Different types of meats generally contribute to a variety of flavors; however the healthiest type is the one with as much lean meat content as possible. Its undisputed fact that the meats that contain a good amount of fat are a culinary treat indeed but for health purposes taking the time to understand the benefits of consuming lean meats is very wise indeed.

It is now common knowledge that nuts greatly help in keeping a lot of ailments in check or from occurring at all. For instance, nuts have been known to be able to keep the possibility of coronary heart diseases manifesting, even for those whole come from a long line of family members with this problem.

Consuming nuts like almonds and walnuts have been known to lower serum cholesterol concentrations within the body system. Nuts are also highly recommended for those individuals suffering from insulin resistance problems like diabetics.

Turning to nuts rather that junk food to quell cravings is also another healthier alternative. Containing essential fatty acids is also another plus point when it comes to choosing nuts as a healthier alternative. Because nuts are healthy and can be consumed in its raw form, it is also another added advantage to keeping these around and handy as snacks.

Almonds are often used to normalize blood lipids because of their slow burn characteristics, which help to keep the blood sugar levels consistently healthy. Rich in a varied amount of different nutrients the almond is a popular additive to the stale diet of most Mediterranean people.

The Brazil nut is also another nutritious nut which comes with its own set of benefits when consumed in moderation. Noted for its omega-3 fatty acid content, the Brazil nut is also a good source of calcium.

Cashew nut is another very popular nut that is often consumed as a salted snack. However it would be a much healthier food product without the addition of salt, as it is already quite a flavorful nut on its own. In some parts of the world these nuts are made into oils.

The selection process should be done with a little knowledge as depending solely on what the naked eye perceives is not enough. Generally lean meats derived from beef cuts should include round, chuck, sirloin and tenderloin, while the cuts from pork or lamb would constitute tenderloin, loin chops and leg. The leanest parts of the poultry would be the breast area without the skin.

Though there are many reasons people eliminate meat from their daily diet, there is no evidence to show that this is a good or bad choice not should it be followed by all.

However the important point to note here is the choice of the types of meats that would make the consumption healthy and this would generally mean meats with lesser amount of fat content.

Though white meat is by no means lacking in fat content, it is by comparison much less in fat content than red meats.

The nutritional value of consuming lean meats is quite extensive and rounded. Lean meats have a generally higher and purer content of protein which is a very important contributing factor to fundamental structural and functional progress of every cell sustenance and formation.

Lean meats are also a good source of essential amino acids particularly sulphur amino acids. When compared to the digestive rates the proteins in meats work faster than the one contained in the beans and whole wheat range.

Lean meat is also a good source of iron. Because iron deficiency is progressive it is often not detected until a later stage where anemia has developed.

Chapter 4- Eating for Different Reasons

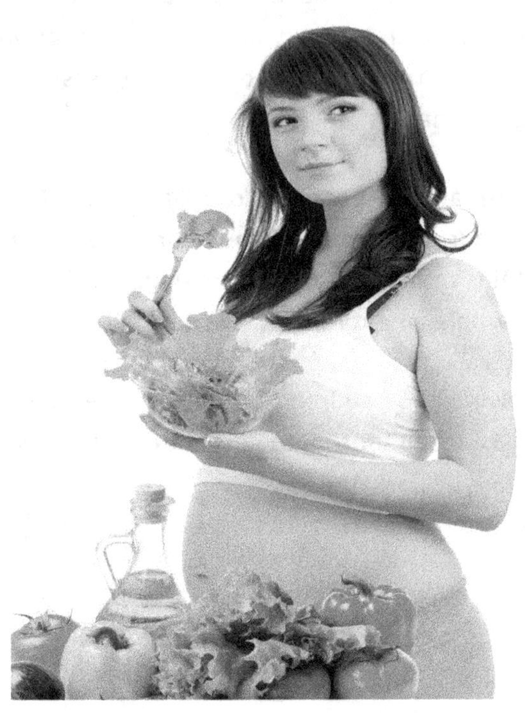

• **To Stimulate Your Passion**

Did you ever sit back and think why your sex life is not so healthy? There could be many reasons. However, did you know that unhealthy eating habits also could be one of the reasons? If you want to have a real healthy and ongoing love/sex life, eating healthy and good food can help you. You want your love life to be strong, regardless of your age, so to make this happen, it is essential that you eat the right kind of food and exercise regularly. This will improve your vigor and stamina.

It is a wrong notion people have that only non-vegetarian food provides lot of strength and not vegetarian food. Well, vegetarian food is also essential to keep your body fit as non-vegetarian food, and can replace non-vegetarian food without any nutritional imbalances in your body. A study has revealed that tomatoes are good for men as it increases their sperm counts.

Chocolates are good foods for females to increase their sex drive. Many foods can improve and maintain a healthy love life, and liver is one such. Some people hate onions because their breath smells. One good way is to reschedule when you eat them, since onions are a great food to improve their sex life. Onions are proven the best sex arousal foods for both men and women.

There are always alternatives to get rid of foul breath, like brushing teeth before going to bed, using mouthwash and chewing on gums. Some people do not eat seafood, but they do not know how seafood especially oysters, which can help them have a fit love life especially have a weak sex life. The most essential part about healthy eating and having a happy sex life is eating the right kind of food and at the right time.

A good breakfast, a healthy lunch, and a light dinner should be a diet program for a normal, fit person. Fruits are other important additions that determine your health. Avoid eating too many bananas, especially if you are a person slightly on the heavier side. Whereas other fruits such as oranges, apples, and watermelon is very health giving. Do not forget to eat carrots and cucumbers. Avoid too much caffeine and alcoholic drinks, as these build fat in your body and decrease your stamina, thus affecting your love life.

Studies show that men and women with low stamina cannot enjoy a healthy sex life. In some countries, people consume a glass of milk before they make love. This helps them get a good arousal and orgasm as well. No matter what age group you belong to, make sure you consult your doctor, if any of the above-recommended food products cause you indigestion or uneasiness. Make sure you eat the right food at the right time. Follow these tips and have a happy love life.

- **To Remain as Healthy Adults**

Most American and European adults face obesity and health related problems. With changing lifestyles, adults fail to pay attention to their nutritional needs. We eat either too much or too little. We are malnourished. A majority of us loses that perfect balance of diet and proper eating habits in the competitive world, where our focus is towards greater earnings. This has affected our lives, and filled it with physical stress and mental pressures. It is high time now that we all give healthy eating first priority and spend our time in better living.

Increasing responsibilities requires one to intake more nutritious and healthy food. With so much to do, your body should get all the essential minerals and vitamins, since improper diets lead to weakness, fatigue and stress. Take precautions and have proper meals at the right time, since having very little food will not fulfil the body's needs, leaving you sick and tired. This is a good example and a warning for your kids as you keep telling them repeatedly to eat healthy to keep fit and trim. Some adults, who simply want to grab a burger, a pizza, or any other junk food to fill their stomachs, and sad to say the kids to learn the wrong eating habits. Junk food may curb the hunger, but it does not take care of your body's nutritional needs.

Your body needs proteins, and other essential minerals to stay fit. Junk food takes away all the vitamins and adds extra saturated fats. This leads to obesity, a sure indicator of health related problems. If you are not healthy, what will you do with your wealth? Unhealthy eating makes your body falls prey to health related problems; you cannot enjoy life and would keep feeling stressed and weak. It is important to spare time to eat, and the time is now. Have small, but healthy meals at regular intervals. Whether you want to lose or gain weight, you must make breakfast the first meal of the day.

Starving does not make you lose weight, and your body runs short of required amounts of nutrients. Consult a dietician and plan your daily diet, which you will follow, of course, if you want a healthy life. Proper food intake at proper times will keep you energetic all day long, and you can carry on with your activities without feeling stressed. When you are well nourished, your brain gets sharp and more alert and you perform well at work and home. You are able to manage life better than before. If they have a proper diet, women do not need to spend on expensive creams and lotions to get the glow on their faces. Keep eating healthy and that glow will stay with you always. Healthy food items revitalize your body systems, helping you lead a healthy and active life.

A proper diet and good exercise keeps many diseases at bay. If the body gets, what it requires, the immune system gets stronger fighting all the unhealthy problems. Even if you fall ill by chance, the immune system helps you recover faster. It is never too late to realize the facts about healthy eating to healthy living. You can start with a proper diet right now and see the difference for yourself. So, the next time you walk in the market do not forget to grab all healthy food for healthy eating.

• For a Healthy Pregnancy

Pregnancy is the time when a woman's body demands more nutrition than ever. As the development and growth of the fetus depends on what you eat, you have to be careful with your eating habits. If you and your baby are deprived of essential proteins and minerals, there can be fatal incidents in the future. For a pregnant woman, it is very important to stick to doctor's advice and follow the diet that well suits needs of a pregnant woman.

Do not fear weight gain, so do not eat less, but do not overeat either. You can always work out and shed the extra pounds later. Never skip meals, and eat after two-hourly intervals. Take in heavy breakfast that includes cereals, fruits, milk, and any other healthy food item. Eat in moderate but let there be more number of meals. Eat lots of green vegetables, small portion of chicken, fish, beans, cheese, peanut butter, dried fruits, juices, soups, skimmed milk, or other dairy products. Every food that you eat should be rich in vitamins, proteins, and minerals but avoid foods that cause allergic reactions. If you have been a junk food addict, avoid it completely as it can affect your baby.

Eat what your body carves for. Being pregnant does not mean you overeat, but eat as much you feel like. However, make sure there is not much of gap in your meals and snacks, as your body will constantly need nutrition's for baby's growth. Be sensibly when you make a choice in food. Being irresponsible towards your diet can cause your baby problems, and an underdeveloped baby is always difficult to take care of. When you are pregnant, do not give up exercise.

Exercise does not mean you hit the gym and do your cardio or weights. Let there be some light exercises. Go on a walk or follow the exercise that your doctor has asked you to follow. Being stiff and not moving around much can cause you difficulty at the time of delivery and thus it is important to let your body do some physical activity. Always take a walk in fresh air so that you and your baby get fresh oxygen to breath.

Drink plenty of water and keep your body hydrated. Take liquids in the form of soups or fruit juices or protein shakes. Drink plenty of water, as it flushes out toxins from your body. It is good to enjoy every meal and do not eat anything that causes your baby discomfort. Certain foods can be a problem, so check with your doctor what to eat and what not to.

Pregnancy is a very sensitive period, and you need to be cautious enough to make sure you and your baby stay in good health. Pregnancy is the time when you eat for two and thus you need to be careful with your choice of food. Maintain a healthy diet throughout your pregnancy, and even after the delivery, to recover faster. Eating healthy will ensure good development of baby, which is important for further growth.

- **To Do Better During Exams**

Did you know that your diet during your exams could determine your performance and success in the exams? Sources have proven that students eating regular and healthy breakfast accomplish better in exams and studies, as compared to those, who miss the most important meal of the day, breakfast. During their exams, students are physically inactive, but still need lots of vitamins, minerals, and iron to concentrate and remember what they read and learn. Lack of any of these can cause adverse effects on the student's performance in studies and exams.

If you feel tired and lazy to study during your exams, this is an indication of low iron and vitamin B content in the body, and can cause deficiency symptoms like paleness, lack of concentration, feeling giddy, etc. To increase your body's iron and vitamin B, both vegetarian and non-vegetarian foods help. Eat vegetarian food like cereals, baked beans, peas, and spinach, and non-vegetarian food like white meat products.

Fish is an important part of the diet because it contains vitamin B, C and E. These vitamins are essential for memory and keep you relaxed. While you have non-veg products, avoid foods that build up body fats. Many students drink tea or coffee while reading or studying, to keep them awake and alert. Well, wake up to the fact that these do not keep you awake. In fact, excess caffeine in the body builds fats and makes you more lethargic.

Drink soups and milk while you study, as they are healthy drinks. Keep tea and coffee to minimum. 1 or 2 cups a day is a good deal. Small meals at regular intervals is not a bad idea, therefore, it is ideal to have 5-7 small meals a day. This keeps your stomach busy and your brain working. One must never miss on fruits, while in the process of studying. For all the essentials that a body needs, fruits are the ultimate choice.

Fruits maintain the sugar level needed by a body through their natural sugar content. Bananas help in increasing weight, oranges helps in building vitamin C, grapes maintain the sugar level, watermelon restrains water-loss from the body and apples provides starch, which indeed gives sugar to the body as natural energy. These are few examples of how important fruits are in a regular diet. Many people do not drink enough water, while studying, because of ignorance or being engrossed in studies. This is wrong, as you must keep yourself hydrated, while you study. Water, juices and soups at regular intervals during the day are good. It is advisable to take a small walk around your house or compound, to help your body digest food properly and fast.

Do not sit down to study immediately after eating as it might make you sleepy and sluggish. If you are a heavy eater, make sure you exercise after eating and then sit to study, in order to refrain from putting on excess weight, and to remain awake during study.

• To Perform Well at Work

With high work pressure and increasing stress levels, most employees barely get time to think about their diet or to follow a health regime. We all know that to survive in this competitive environment, you have to go that extra mile to get noticed at your work place. But that does not mean you have to compromise with your health. There are many ways, you can ensure your calorie and vitamin intake is sufficient for the whole day.

Firstly, it is important to have breakfast, before you leave home. This is the most essential meal of the day, as it provides you with vigor for the whole day. For workingwomen, it is very important to have milk for breakfast, and a combination of milk with oats or low calorie cornflakes is ideal, as it is easy to make and provides you with calcium and the essential nutrients. If you have the time, you can also boil an egg and eat, as it will provide you with enough protein and cut out the carbohydrates. While you are at work, you are bound to be tempted to have several cups of coffee, but avoid this temptation.

A cup of coffee a day does not harm you, but once you start having more than a cup a day, your calorie intake due to sugar and caffeine intake increases body weight much faster. You may have too much work piled up at office, you may be in a meeting, or you may be just too consumed with work, to realize you have skipped a meal or what you are eating is absolutely unhealthy.

The first rule is to choose your food wisely. If you are in a meeting and you have been served working lunch, don't stuff yourself with the cheese pizzas and sandwiches. Instead, go for the salads or pizzas with more green. Instead of Coke, ask for water or a fruit juice. Make it a point to be one of those people who can eat what they have brought from home, and on time. Make yourself a salad with a few chicken cubes and with low fat salad topping. If you need bread make sure, it's brown. This type of meal is high in fiber and protein and helps you control, even lose weight.

After you get home, you tend to indulge in a snack, and so you tend to eat either fried or sweet food. Keep reminding yourself that you have not indulged in any strenuous physical activity and you can always supplement the snack with fruits or even some refreshing juice and a few biscuits. Lastly, remember to have an early dinner rich in protein that includes meat and leafy vegetables to give you an ideal diet for the whole day. And most importantly, remember to get at least 45 minutes of exercise, five days a week to keep your body in good shape and stay fit.

- **To Maintain Youth and Vigor**

Today's youth spend a hell of a lot on expensive creams and lotions to restore and maintain their beauty. The question is how many are successful in getting the glow on their face? If you do not follow a healthy diet, no cream or lotion will ever help you look young or make you feel good. You look what you eat, and thus, to look younger than your age, and feel fresh and energetic throughout the day, take care of your eating habits.

If you meet any beautiful woman whose age looks the same for years together, make it a point do ask them the secret behind it. Believe me, they will tell you that the way to healthy skin and youthful looks are healthful foods, not any branded creams. To feel good and look young, change your diet. Putting yourself in to a habit of eating healthy is the best solution for all your health problems. Consult a dietician for advice on types of food intake you should follow.

Due to their busy schedules, many people complain that they get no time to eat regular meals. However, food should be your first priority especially when you have a busy schedule. Kick-start your day with a heavy and nutritious breakfast for more energy to go about your daily activities. Cereals make a good breakfast. Replace white bread to brown break and feel the difference. Drink a glass of juice or milk as per your choice. Add lots of leafy vegetables to your diet. Salads provide you with all necessary vitamins. A fruit after every meal is great and enhances your energy levels. When having meat, make sure you go for lean meat. This keeps a check on your fat levels.

Fish is a good source of omega 3 fatty acid, and you should certainly include fish in your diet. Beans, nuts, and eggs are high on proteins that are required for the body development. Do not completely cut down on fats as your body needs some percentage for the growth and development. You can choose low fats food stuff to control the body fats. A balanced diet makes sure you are high on energy levels, and makes you feel peppy all day long. The results that you get from healthy food items, no other artificial food item can give.

Natural food items have all the minerals and essential vitamins that make you feel good and look naturally young. With healthy eating habits, you never have to worry about any side effects or other healthy related problems. Keep yourself away from artificial juices and junk food. When in restaurants, learn to select your dishes properly. It is good to keep your temptation in control and order healthy and nutritious food.

There is no reason to get bored with healthy food items, as you can experiment with your cooking. You can try various dishes and cook in different styles to make it look appetizing. All it takes a great deal to put yourself in the habit of healthy eating, it is worth it in the long run. It is never too late to start eating healthy as it has lots of benefits for all.

- **For a Better Heart**

Records of medical related deaths in the last few decades show that the most number related to cardiac arrests, and heart related problems. Being a crucial part of the body, and you should take care to keep your heart healthy. People go usually for taste and not for quality of food. They overlook foods that give them energy nutrients, and opt for foods that give taste, and kill hunger. Almost everyone eats at fast food joints that serve junk, but which tastes yummy. Have you ever realized how much damage burgers, fries, sausages, and other fast food causes to the heart? Consumption of excess salt and sugar is also considered unhealthy for the heart. Yes, it is very difficult to keep away from those tempting delicious hamburgers and juicy sausages. However, make sure you keep away from them or get prepared to face a round of heart stopping trouble. The only alternative to a hamburger is no hamburger, but if you must, ensure that they contain very little mayonnaise, and the sausages stir fried in low amounts of refined oil. Studies show that about 80% of heart diseases can be reduced through healthy and proper diet.

Well, if you are one of those people that eating fattening foods and have oodles of excess weight, it's high time you control your diet and follow the following tips.

Vegetarian foods:

There is nothing as healthy as pure vegetarian food. It is not that vegetarian foods don't contain fats. They do, but less. Green leafy vegetables, carrots, tomatoes, cucumbers are considered very healthy and adds no cholesterol to your body.

Non-vegetarian foods:

There are a few methods to cook non-veg foods to reduce the cardiac risk. Add spice to your non-veg foods by mixing sage, dill, dry mustard, marjoram, tarragon, oregano, garlic, onions etc., as these reduce cholesterol and fat saturation.

Extra activities:

Smoking, alcohol, excess caffeine in the body can also add to the risk of heart diseases. In order to keep your heart healthy, reduce or eliminate these from your life, and be involved in regular physical exercises that include cycling, running, jogging, cross training, etc. All this, not only makes your cardio-vascular system strong, but also builds your stamina. Here's a list of both vegetarian and non- vegetarian foods that can help you remain fit and keep your heart healthy:

White meat, lean red meat, wholegrain foods, green/red fruits and vegetables, low fat milk and milk products, and low cholesterol oil or olive oil. Eat low saturated fat foods and carefully read the ingredients used in your food and do not trust the labels saying low cholesterol. Chocolates, fast/junk foods, mayonnaise, cheese, butter, etc. should be avoided as much as possible.

Remember; avoid Low-Density Lipoprotein (LDL), which is bad cholesterol, as it causes heart complexities; whereas High-Density Lipoprotein (HDL) is the good cholesterol, which should be present in the body to prevent cardio vascular risks. Things like heredity, gender and age cannot be controlled, but things that affect them can surely be. Hence, eating healthy food and keeping a watch over your diet would better keep your heart safe.

CHAPTER 5- HOW TO EAT HEALTHY ANYTIME, ANYWHERE

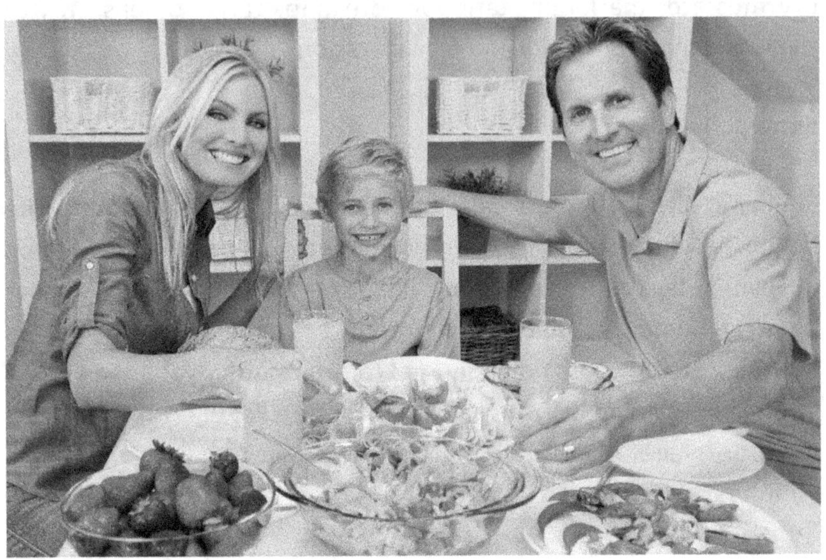

- **When in a Restaurant**

If you have started eating healthy food at home, then you need to extend it while dining out, since a single high-fat or high-calorie meal can undo your entire week's hard work. A little research and a little care while dining out will result in eating food that not only tastes good, but is also light in calories. Narrow down restaurants that do not serve greasy or oily food or those that at least offers a healthier version of their regular food. You should inquire if the restaurant is willing to provide grilled or lightly sautéed dishes, instead of just frying them.

Restaurants that serve different cuisines such as Italian, Mexican, American, Chinese, and Indian require different approaches. But, as a general rule of thumb, ensure that your intake of fresh vegetables in the form of salads or other side dishes is quite high. This ensures that you do not wolf down only on meat or pizzas topped with double cheese.

The key to dining out is to savor the fine taste of various dishes. Instead of concentrating on only one item, try to eat smaller servings of various dishes. This will please your palette, while ensuring that you do not concentrate on a single high-calorie dish. Order a salad sprinkled with lime, salt and pepper instead of one doused with mayonnaise. Even while trying sauce-based dishes, eat those that have a tomato base instead of a cream base.

Avoid drinking sweetened carbonated sodas, and instead drink tea or coffee sweetened with sugar substitutes, or better still drink fresh fruit juices or water. Avoid soups that have a lot of cream content and instead stick to clear soup or tomato soup. A soup will dull your appetite and so, you will not eat too much. Try not to finish the entire dish at one go, but instead get some of it packed to re-heat the next day. If at a fast-food restaurant, order a single-patty burger that has only dry salad instead of cheese and mayonnaise. Even pizzas should be thin crust or whole wheat based with less cheese and high vegetable toppings, instead of a thick crust double cheese pizza with red meat topping. In short, substitute any dish that is dripping with molten cheese or butter with one that only has a little cheese or butter spread thinly over it.

By cutting down on high-fat and high-calorie dishes, you will still enjoy your meal without piling on the unwanted calories to your body. Order one dessert and share it with your partner; this is a good way to control your calorie intake. You can thus keep a watch on the quality of food you eat, when you dine out and a little care and research goes a long way to make your dining experience memorable and filling, without having a negative effect on your health.

- **When under Stress**

Stress is an unavoidable companion, of nearly every urbanite in this fast paced world. A high stress level may force you into an unhealthy eating cycle, which could further complicate your health. On the other hand, eating healthy food could actually help you to reduce your stress levels and helps you bounce into this high stress arena with aplomb.

Work pressures might lead to building stress levels up, and these results in low energy levels, fatigue and often with a feeling of depression. Pressure of time might force you to eat unhealthy fast food over a longer period. This results in starving your body of vital vitamins, proteins and carbohydrates essential to power your body and mind. So, stop buying your food from fast food pick-ups, and instead substitute it with healthy alternatives that can be prepared in a jiffy. So, instead of picking up donuts, burgers, or pizzas, pick up fruit, and fruit juices without preservatives, or sandwiches made of whole wheat bread or cookies made of whole wheat.

Synthetically prepared fast foods provide only temporary relief by spiking sugar levels. Trans-fat and cholesterol rich food, instead of helping your body and mind, only end up weakening the body's immune system. This cycle will continue until your body or your mind eventually breaks down. But, if you start eating the right foods, you could soon refresh your body and mind and this will enable you keep the stress causing demons at bay.

A healthy breakfast of eggs, grilled bacon, whole wheat bread or cookies with fresh fruit juice or even bananas blended in cold milk does not require a lot of preparation time, yet tastes extremely good. Lunch could consist of pastas or rice noodles with your choice of fresh vegetables, which should not be fried, but lightly sautéed or just boiled. Salads made of various vegetables and fruits are also a healthy option and provide a tasty side dish. If you do not find the time to make a salad, then you could just have a tasty vegetable juice. Sandwiches made of granary bread with a variety of fillings like vegetables, lightly grilled white meat, or egg white also make for a healthy lunch. You can add butter or cheese to your sandwiches, but remember to stay in calorific control.

For those in-between snacks, keep natural canned fruit or whole-wheat crackers or cookies in your office or store. Try to restrict your tea or coffee intake to two cups in a day and replace them with lemon juice or any other vegetable juice of your choice. Make sure to rotate your vegetables, fruits and salads, in order to stay motivated and not get bored within a short time. In order to suppress any untoward cravings, you can eat burgers, chocolates and pizzas occasionally, but ensure that it does not turn into a regular habit, again. Instead of eating the wrong kind of food that only add to your stress problems, ensure that you follow a healthy food regime that in fact helps you to fight stress and also ensures that you keep stress away in future.

- **Before a Big Game**

With the Big Game around the corner, the first thing a player needs to keep in mind is to stay lean and fit. Regular exercises and a healthy diet keep a player in the best of shape to play that all-important game, but playing the Big Game adds its own level of physical and mental strengths. There are specific exercises to do and foods that an athlete or player can consume to gain stamina and strength.

One of the important parts of gaining muscle is definitely to exercise. Apart from this, regular protein intake is necessary to give the body its required strength and help build muscles. Necessary amount of protein supplements are a quick and easy way to get nourishment, but not recommended. Protein-rich meals can be consumed every day, avoiding unnecessary spending on protein supplements.

Always remember excess of anything is not good. Few people go a step ahead and take in excess protein, which is only stored as extra energy or fat. Before your game, eat a low fat meal with enough proteins and carbohydrates and give at least 2 hours for your stomach to digest the food. When you know your game will last for more than an hour, ensure you consume meals with lots of carbohydrates 2 to 3 days before your game. This ensures that muscles store more carbohydrates, and gives you higher endurance during your long game.

An ideal diet break up of calories for sportsmen is, approximately 60% of carbohydrates, 20% protein and 20% fat. After practicing and sweating, replace your body's depleted salts and minerals. You can do so with your regular meals, lime juice or glucose. Make sure all bodily minerals are replaced, as you don't want to get dehydrated. Ignoring thirst after a long hard game can lead to cramps as well. So make sure all bodily fluids are replenished in due time. The next question that will arise is what are the ideal sources of vitamins, minerals, proteins, carbohydrates etc.?

To give you a brief description of each source of nutrients:

•For the right amount of vitamins and minerals, each meal should contain bright colored vegetables like carrots, spinach, and pepper.

•To get an adequate amount of calcium, milk and all dairy products are the best option.

•For iron, you should eat chicken, tuna, and leafy green vegetables.

•For a good amount of protein, go for fish, chicken, soy products, and nuts.

•Fibrous food such as wheat or pasta is rich in carbohydrates. Sportsmen should eat this to acquire adequate amount of energy to be stored in the muscles.

•Lastly, to replenish your body of all vitamins and salts lost due to sweating, water is the best option. The ideal amount would be 1 cup of water, after every twenty to thirty minutes of exercise.

While a few sportsmen maintain a balanced diet, some concentrate on burning calories and losing weight, so, when you need to excel, ensure that you get the right amounts of all nutrients to excel.

• **When Travelling**

While travelling by road, rail, air or sea, you might find that your choice of eating healthy food is severely curtailed. The main reason is that most joints that dish out food to travelers concentrate more on their turnover of food rather than ensuring that the dish has the right calories and nutrition. So, it depends on you to locate and choose the dish that not only satisfies your taste buds, but also provides the right fuel for your body.

The basic problem in eating healthy food during travelling is that you might tend to lose control over food, which may be due to eating home-made food for a long time or if you lay your eyes on some local delicacies along the way. If you cannot resist the temptation of trying out various delicacies along the way, then at least try to limit the quantity by sharing the dish with your loved ones. In addition, try to have items with less calories and more nutritional value, and are light on the stomach. If you are travelling by road and need to have your breakfast at a small service station, then do not order fried bacon or deep fried eggs in any form. Instead, order for a sandwich or cereals with hot or cold milk. In case you order eggs ensure that you stick to boiled eggs or an omelet with lightly buttered toast.

Ensure that you and your children eat nutritious snacks along the way. Instead of eating French fries or chips that have high salt and fat levels, pack whole wheat bread with peanut butter or cheese slices and protein bars along with fresh fruits or fruit juices. Avoid coffee and tea. Assorted nuts such as walnuts and cashews make for good in-between snacks. These food items will keep your children busy and will also save a lot of money along the way. Check the road map and try to locate any other restaurants along the way, where you can get access to healthy food. Ensure that you choose the right salads and fillings, since not all the ingredients are low in calories. Even if you are travelling by train, plane, or ship, try to do a mental calculation of the calories and check out the positive and negative aspects of any dish, before ordering it. Try sticking to baked, boiled or roasted dishes instead of fried ones.

If you are having lunch along the way, then go in for a light soup followed by dishes containing white meat instead of red meat. Ensure that you have adequate side dishes containing vegetables or salads to complement your meat dish. The key to eating healthy during travelling is to avoid the temptation of stuffing yourself along the way. You should eat food that keeps you alert and thus enables you to enjoy your travel, instead of making you sluggish. By keeping an eye out for healthy food and sticking to your resolution of eating only sensible food, you can enjoy your journey, while remaining healthy at the same time.

• After a Night of Drinking

If you have had a night filled with fun, dance, and lots of drinks, then you could wake up with a pounding head and a mouth that might have suddenly turned to coarse sand paper. Alcohol can rob the body of vital nutrients including sugar and so it is vital to get the right ingredients back into your body to not only limit the effects of your overnight hangover, but also get back in physical and mental shape, if you want to enjoy the day after.

In order to limit the effects of a hangover, drink lots of water between your drinks, even if it reduces the buzz. This will definitely reduce the hangover by flushing out the alcohol from your system. You need to realize that your body is severely dehydrated due to excessive alcohol and in case you start your morning by drinking coffee or any other products containing caffeine, you could only make the situation go from bad to ugly. In addition to sugar, alcohol also drains away your magnesium and potassium levels.

A healthy breakfast is what can actually get you back on your wobbly feet in no time. Even though you might not feel hungry during a hangover, it is important to eat a full breakfast, since even though your mind might not be willing; your body actually needs the vital vitamins, salt and sugar to start functioning again. Traditional breakfast items like baked beans, bacon, and eggs in various forms can help out a lot. You can also replenish lost vitamins by slowly sipping a glass of orange juice.

The important point is to eat slowly, since a heavy breakfast after a heavy night can result in your stomach revolting and throwing everything out, thus resulting in even more hangover problems. Instead of frying everything, try to grill, so that your breakfast remains healthy and the chances of throwing up get reduced. You could also eat bananas to recover the lost potassium levels or if you can arrange for some natural coconut water, then that could be even better since it has more potassium levels than bananas.

Do not try to eat or drink anything new, but instead stick to foods that your body is already adapted to, if you do not want any complications. Also, ensure that you drink adequate water and juice throughout the day. If the prospect of a heavy breakfast is unappealing, then try to have a banana smoothie along with some pieces of toast made of whole wheat bread. This could be light on your stomach and you could have another heavy breakfast of bacon, beans or eggs after a couple of hours. It is better to ignore advice to drink wine or any other alcoholic drink as a cure, since even though it might offer temporary relief by keeping you in a state of suspended high, ultimately your body will pay a higher price, since it will only result in increased dehydration. You will only end up delaying your hangover, instead of eliminating it.

Try to stay away from tea and coffee, since caffeine again will only give you temporary mental relief, but will actually dehydrate your body further. A shower will also help you to get fresh. A little bit of care before, during and after an enjoyable drinking night can thus negate most of the harmful effects of a hangover. Eating and drinking the above-mentioned foods, fruits and drinks is thus a healthy and quick way to bounce back on your feet and can also help to clear your mind to face the coming day.

- **During the Holidays**

When the holidays arrive, many people forget all about their diets and healthy eating. Weight gains of 7 to 10 pounds are common between Halloween and Christmas. To make the holidays easier, these tips will help you with healthy eating through the season and not gaining weight.

Most traditional foods can be made low fat. Turkey is very lean without the skin, and gravy can be made without any fat. Potatoes that are served without butter can be very healthy. The beloved pumpkin pie is nutritious, although it can be made into a fatty dessert with the adding of whipped cream.

Even though the holidays are in, don't forget about the exercise. You should plan a walk after meals, park farther from stores when you shop, and take a few walks around the mall before you begin shopping.

During holiday parties and at family dinners, feel free to sample foods although you shouldn't splurge. Decide on what you plan to eat in advance, and then stick to your plan. Eat plenty of vegetables, fruit, low fat dressings, and slices of lean meats. Before you go to a party, eat a small snack to help curb your appetite.

If at all possible, avoid alcohol. Having too many drinks can cripple your will power, and also add excess calories to your diet. In the place of alcohol, drink water with lemon. Water can help to limit your appetite and keep you from bingeing. Also make sure to avoid eggnog, as each glass can have up to 300 calories.

Be flexible with your healthy eating, as one bad meal will not ruin your diet. Try to balance your calories over a few days and don't just look at one meal or day.

CHAPTER 6- THE HEALTHIEST FOODS

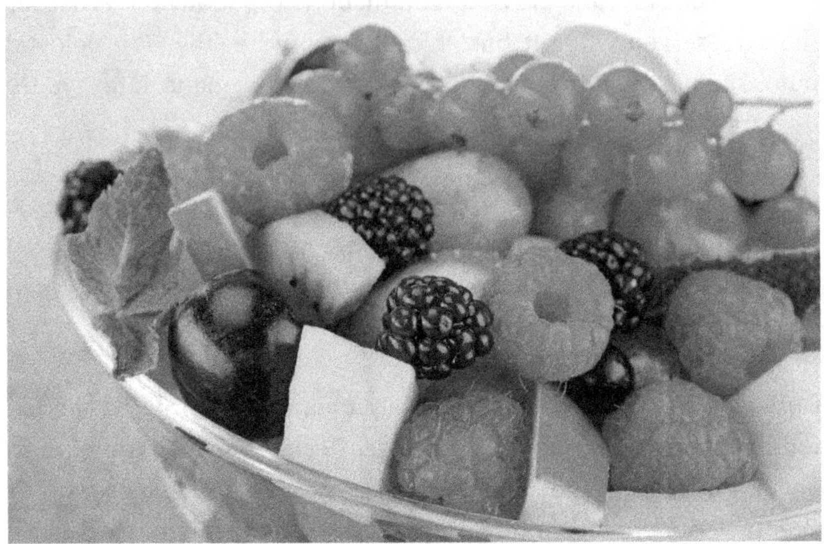

The following is a list of the healthiest foods that you can get. This will help you get an idea as to what foods are the best for your body.

Fruits

Apricots: Apricots contain Beta-carotene which helps to prevent radical damage and also helps to protect the eyes. A single apricot contains 17 calories, 0 fat, and one gram of fiber. You can eat them dried or soft.

Mango: A medium sized mango packs 57 MG of vitamin C, which is nearly your entire daily dose. This antioxidant will help prevent arthritis and also boost your immune system.

Cantaloupe: Cantaloupes contain 117 GG of vitamin C, which is almost twice the recommended dose. Half a melon contains 853 MG of potassium, which is nearly twice as much as a banana, which helps to lower blood pressure. Half a melon contains 97 calories, 1 gram of fat, and 2 grams of fiber.

Tomato: A tomato can help cut the risk of bladder, stomach, and colon cancers in half if you eat one daily. A tomato contains 26 calories, 0 fat, and only 1 gram of fiber.

Vegetables

Onions: An onion can help to protect against cancer. A cup of onions offers 61 calories, 0 fat, and 3 grams of fiber.

Broccoli: Broccoli can help protect against breast cancer, and it also contains a lot of vitamin C and beta- carotene. One cup of chopped broccoli contains 25 calories, 0 fat, and 3 grams of fiber.

Spinach: Spinach contains carotenoids that can help fend off macular degeneration, which is a major cause of blindness in older people. One cup contains 7 calories, 0 fat, and 1 gram of fiber.

Grains, beans, and nuts

Peanuts: Peanuts and other nuts can lower your risk of heart disease by 20 percent. One ounce contains 166 calories, 14 grams of fat, and over 2 grams of fiber.

Pinto beans: A half cup of pinto beans offers more than 25 percent of your daily folate requirement, which protects you against heart disease. Half a cup contains 103 calories, 1 gram of fat, and 6 grams of fiber.

Skim milk: Skim milk offers vitamin B2, which is important for good vision and along with Vitamin A, could improve allergies. You also get calcium and vitamin D as well. One cup contains 86 calories, 0 fat, and 0 fiber.

Seafood

Salmon: All cold water fish such as salmon, mackerel, and tuna are excellent sources of omega 3 fatty acids, which help to reduce the risk of cardiac disease. A 3 ounce portion of salmon contains 127 calories, 4 grams of fat and 0 fiber.

Crab: Crab is a great source of vitamin B12 and immunity boosting zinc. A 3 ounce serving of crab offers 84 calories, 1 gram of fat and 0 fiber.

How to Read Nutrition Labels

The nutrition label located on each and every food item, will tell you all the information about that food. For some, however, this information isn't exactly that reader friendly. Fear not, as it's actually easier than you think.

Serving Size

This size is based on the amount people eat. Similar food items will have similar serving sizes, thus making it easier to compare 2 foods of the same category.

% Daily Value

This indicates how food will fit in a 2,000 calorie diet. This will help you to understand if the food has a lot, or just a little of the important nutrients.

The Middle Section

The nutrients you'll find listed in the middle section are the ones that are most important to your health. This information can help you to calculate your daily limit of fat, fiber, sodium, and other nutrients.

Vitamins & Minerals

The percent daily value found here is the exact same as the U.S. Recommended Daily Allowance for vitamins and minerals.

Now that you know what the nutrition label actually means, it'll be a lot easier to eat healthy. Eating healthy is a great thing - especially when you use the nutrition label to assist you with your food choices.

Chapter 7- Planning Healthier Meals on a Budget

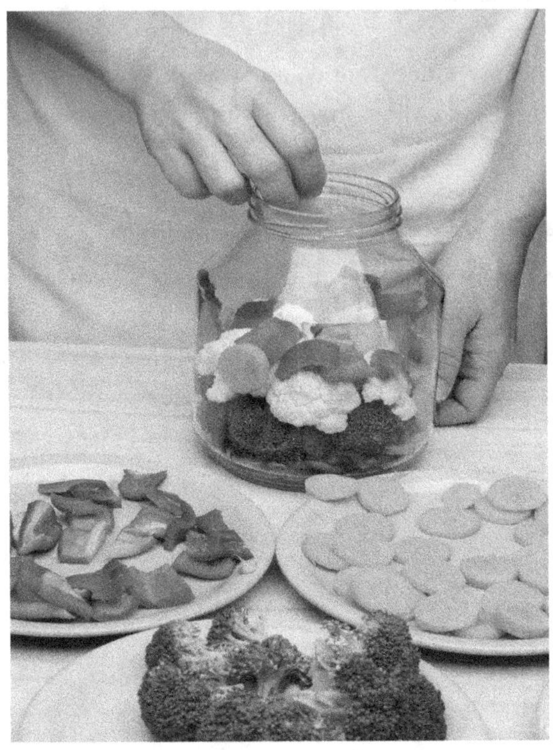

If you have problems serving healthy foods because of the prices, you'll find these tips to be just what you need to eat healthy on a budget.

1. Eliminate junk food. Doing your shopping on your own is the easiest way to shop, as children and sometimes spouses are usually the ones requesting junk food. Shopping alone will prevent this, and ensure that you only buy the foods you need.

2. Water or milk instead of soft drinks. You can still enjoy your favorite drinks at a sporting event or night out, although you should stick with the smallest size when shopping to save money and calories. Children and even adults need milk or milk products

on a daily basis. Milk will also help you get strong and provides calcium for healthy bones and healthy teeth.

3. Buy fruits in quantity. When they are in season, buy fruits in quantity and freeze any extras. You can buy several pounds this way, and freeze extras to have them when the fruit goes out of season. Wash the fruit well, remove any spoiled pieces, dry thoroughly, and then freeze in plastic zipper bags.

4. Meats and beans. Meats and beans are the best sources for protein. Lean meat is more expensive than meats with a lot of fat.

Canned beans are a great deal as well, as they give you protein at a great price.

5. Beans as a substitute. You should use beans a substitute for meat on a frequent occasion. There are several varieties, so you can prepare them in a crock pot, so when you return home they are ready to consume. The USDA recommends eating beans at least 4 times per week. If you experience gas after eating beans you should try washing them, covering them with water, bringing the water to a boil, then draining it off and refilling the pot.

6. If you live in a coastal area or an area where fish are around, make that an integral part of your diet. You can catch them from the lakes or rivers, saving money in the process.

7. Peanut butter is great for those on a budget as it's popular with almost everyone. You can use it for sandwiches instead of eating hot dogs. It does not need to be refrigerated, and bigger jars can last you for weeks.

8. You should fill up with foods that have a high content of water. Watermelon, salads, and even sugar free gelatin are all great examples.

Eating healthy is always something you can't go wrong with. You can eat healthy for just a few bucks, which makes it perfect for those on a budget.

Now, you don't need a lot of money to have the lifestyle and health you've always wanted.

Become a Smart Shopper

Grocery shopping is something we all have to do, even though choosing the right foods can be very hard indeed. To assist you with your healthy grocery shopping, the tips below can indeed help make things easier than ever before:

1. Never go grocery shopping on an empty stomach.

2. Select canned fruits and tuna that are packed in water, not oil or syrup.

3. Look at the labels for the words "hydrogenated" or "partially hydrogenated". The earlier you see them appear on the list, the higher the amount of unhealthy Trans fatty acids the food will contain.

4. Don't buy turkey with the skin on it, and if you plan to buy chicken - buy a chicken breast.

5. When you select frozen dinners, select those that are not only low in fat, but low in sodium and cholesterol as well.

6. If you are not consuming enough dairy products, go with calcium fortified orange juice instead.

7. Go for whole grain breads, cereals, and rolls.

8. Give cantaloupe a try. With just 95 calories, half of the melon will provide more than a day's supply of Vitamin C and beta carotene.

9. Don't be tricked into buying yogurt covered by nuts or raisins, as the coating is normally made of sugar and partially hydrogenated oils.

10. Get some of the low fat treats, such as pretzels, ginger snaps, and angel food cake.

By following the above tips when grocery shopping, you'll avoid the bad foods and get those that you need. There are many different healthy foods at the grocery store; all it takes is the will power to go past the bad foods and on to the good ones.

Chapter 8- How to Encourage Kids and Teens to Eat Healthy

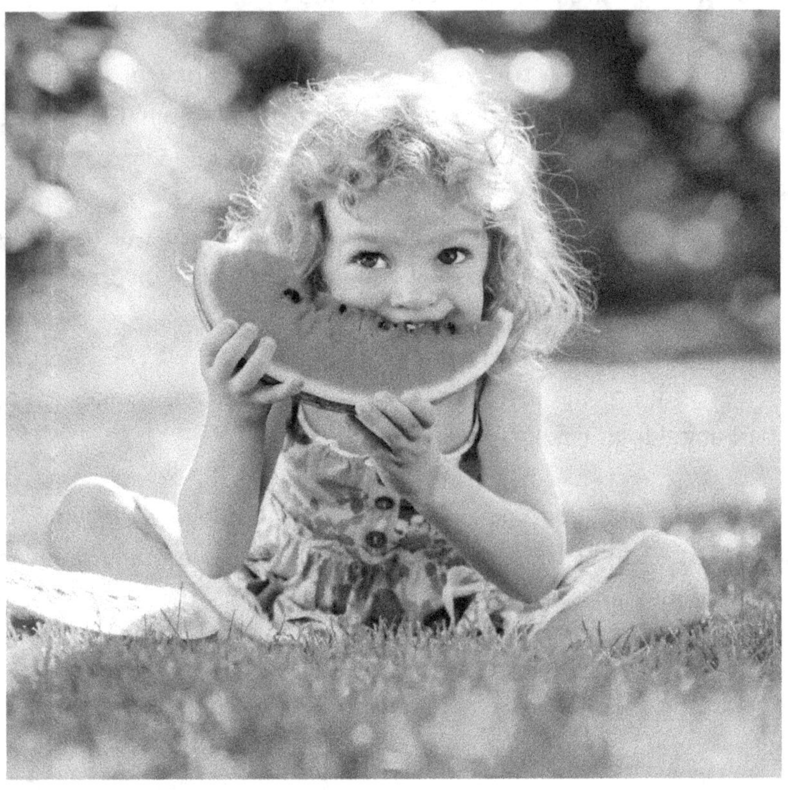

Fast food is a big part of modern life these days, making it very hard to teach a child how he or she should eat healthy. The cheapest and easiest foods are those that are normally the least healthy. If you give your child the choice between healthy food and junk food, you normally will not like the results. Even though it isn't possible to get a child to like all healthy foods, there are some ways to get your child to try and hopefully like at least a few of them. You can be as creative as you like, as getting kids to eat healthy foods can be a little harder than you may think.

- Sneak the healthy food in. Even though it would be great if your kid understood the importance of fruits and vegetables, this isn't always possible. If you can't get them to eat good food willingly, there are ways to sneak them in, such as making muffins out of bananas or apples, or pizza with spinach on it.

- Call fruits and vegetables by funny names. You can refer to broccoli as "trees", making them more fun to eat. There are many different names you can call fruits and vegetables, even making up your own if you prefer. Most kids prefer to eat foods that sound fun.

- Make the foods taste better. Ranch dressing is great for broccoli, while peanut butter is a great topping for celery. There are several combinations for vegetables that can make them taste much better. You can let your child pick a topping for a vegetable; even if it's something you wouldn't normally like yourself.

- Dress the vegetables up. Just as much as calling them names help kids eat healthy foods, making them look funny also helps. You can do this by making funny designs on the plate, or setting them up to look like people. Although some parents don't like their kids playing with their food, sometimes it helps to get them to eat healthier.

There are several ways to make your kids eat healthier, but to make them enjoy it also has to be fun as well. This isn't always an easy task, because kids normally don't like foods that are good for them. It can, however, be done with a bit of creativity. Hopefully, doing this will help your child develop a love of healthy foods for the rest of their lives.

Create Fun Recipes for Kids

A lot of studies and research has shown that kids who eat breakfast perform better in school and have a healthier diet. Eating breakfast will help promote the proper growth and maximize school performance as well. Breakfast is often times a victim of the morning time crunch.

Even though you may be tempted to skip breakfast, you can simplify your morning routine by following these 8 tips:

1. Finish homework and pack school bags at night.

2. Decide on what your children will wear to school before you go to bed and locate lost shoes for the following day.

3. In the morning, get up 15 minutes earlier.

4. Give up computer games and morning television.

5. Have healthy foods on hand. You should also shop for breakfast foods with your kids and take into account their personal preferences.

6. Set the cereal out the night before. For younger children, fill a zippered plastic bag with her portion, then add the milk in the morning.

7. Allow your children to use the microwave often, as most breakfast foods can be prepared in less than 5 minutes.

8. Allow your kids to eat in the car or on the way to school.

There are several foods that you can eat for breakfast, even leftovers from supper if they are sufficient. You can eat bagels, pizza with fruit juice, pretzels, or the normal bacon and eggs that breakfast is known for. Most foods are a snap to prepare, and will not take you but a few minutes.

The next time you are in a hurry in the morning, remember that you are probably about to skip the most important meal of the day. If you follow the tips above, you'll find that you have plenty of time for breakfast.

Teaching Teens to Skip the Junk and Fast Food

Growing children need plenty of energy to perform their daily activities. An average teenager is involved in high intensity activities compared to an office goer. Activities can be low, medium, and high intensity. Study, play, exams, camps, trips, big games, tours, etc., are some of the many activities that form part of a teenager's life through the day. He/she needs both, mental and physical strength up with this routine, to remain fit and healthy.

A teenager's diet of should contain carbohydrates, proteins, minerals, vitamins, and all the essentials that their bodies need. A teenager should have more food as compared to a 45 year old. This is because teenagers have high metabolism rates. Five or six medium meals justify an average teenager's diet pattern. A little bit of fatty food is again not a problem because the fats in the body disappear the moment they start engaging themselves in different games, trips or any other activities. In fact, teenagers should eat heavy meals, as this is their only time to build strong bodies.

How To Be Healthier One Bite At A Time
The essential and healthy food items for a teenager are:

- Milk provides calcium for healthy teeth and bones. Water content in the milk keeps you hydrated.

- Fruit juices give the teenager that little boost in stamina required while they play.

- Water an average teenager must consume at least 8-10 liters of water per day.

- Meat and eggs provides proteins, vitamins and carbohydrates. Very essential to increase weight and muscle mass. Fish helps in increasing concentration and alertness.

- Fruits and vegetables are more essential than non-vegetarian food. It is important because the minerals and vitamins are needed for the body and keeps the body hydrated. Fruits also help in learning and remembering. Dieticians recommend plenty of fruits and vegetables for growing teens. Fruits and vegetables are great to gain weight and remain fit.

All the above food items help teens in their studies and physical activities. The food cycle of an average teenager should be heavy breakfast at about seven, a fruit around 10, good lunch at about one, a fruit at about 3, and a small meal at around 5 with a fruit juice and dinner at 8.

A growing teen must not eat oily or fattening foods, as this might make him/her lazy, lethargic or even build excess body fats, which are the initial stages of obesity. If your teenager is not engaged in sports or exercises, absolutely do not follow the abovementioned foods, since with healthy eating; there should always be good exercise. Teens with low metabolism rate often put on more weight, even if they eat less. This is not correct. The idea is to eat healthy and exercise more to increase the metabolism rate and reduce the unwanted fats in the body.

Teens that are always attached to the computer or are at home should reduce the intake of meat, energy drinks, and milk, as it is not necessary for them and they might put on fats in their bodies. To conclude, teens should stop eating junk food from outside and stick to home cooked food to stay healthy and fit.

Chapter 9- Obesity and Healthy Eating

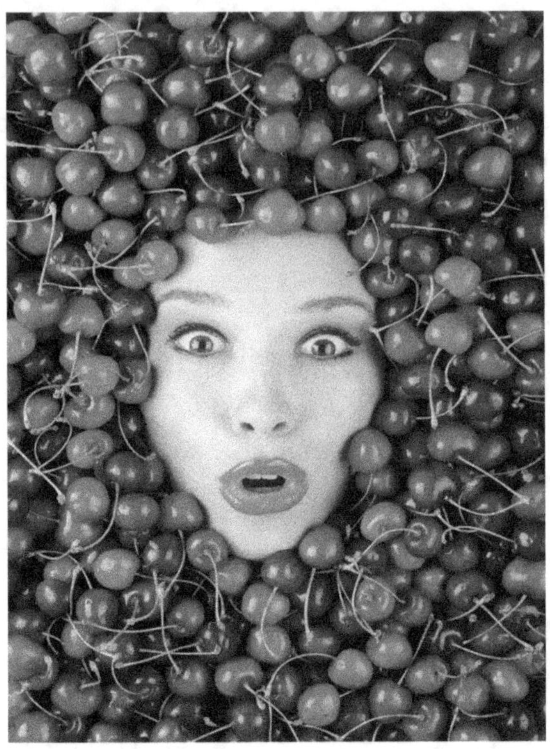

Seeing obese persons has now become a common feature. Every other person is overweight, if not obese. Besides making a person look ungainly, obesity affects a person adversely, posing severe health hazards. There are various reasons for obesity; however, there are no advantages to being obese, only disadvantages. If you are obese and you want to lose that extra body fat, a perfect diet is essential. A diet that is chalked out considering your age, gender, and fat percentage and body weight would be a perfect diet. Visit a dietician, who is an expert in this field and share with him/her your eating habits and lifestyle.

Here are a few tips on how you can start with a fat-loss program, which you could follow yourself.

Diet:

Make a list of dishes that you eat throughout the day for a week. After that, make a note of fatty food that you consume. Consult a dietician to know what contains fat and what is nutritious. Eliminate those items from your list that generate unnecessary fats in your body. If those items are your favorites, reduce their consumption to start with. If you are one of those, who overeat, then you need to have plenty of water just before you start your meal and if you feel hungry after every 2 hours, then try having salads or fruits, and not bananas. There is nothing better than a fruit and vegetable diet. Some of the best foods are boiled vegetables, fruit salads, vegetable salads, etc., which supply vitamins and minerals for the body and make you fit. Breakfast being your first meal of the day should be at about 7 am and must be heavy and nutritious. Lunch should be a little light at about 1 pm and your dinner has to be bare minimum by 7pm. Eating healthy meals on time is necessary for fat loss. Always follow the saying, "eat your breakfast alone, share your lunch with friends and give your dinner to your enemy".

Exercise:

Exercise to lose extra body fats. Your work out should mainly consist of cardio vascular exercises, such as running, jogging, cycling, skipping, etc. Fat loss is the result of balanced combination of diet and exercise. Do not make the mistake of exercising vigorously, initially. Many people get carried away with the whole weight loss spree and end up with severe body pain and miss out on further exercises. If you are used to exercising, you can very well go ahead with your work out and gradually increase exercising more. Here is a tip on how to increase your metabolism rate and lose fats faster. Work out for the biggest muscle of your body, your legs. Consisting of quadriceps, hamstrings and calves, your legs have to be strong and not fat, as they carry your entire weight.

Other things:

Reduce alcohol, aerated drinks, sweets, chocolates, oily foods, and other fattening edibles drastically. They contribute a lot to obesity. Overeating and continuous eating also adds to obesity. Obesity is one of the causes for cardiac arrests in many people. Therefore eat healthy, exercise well and beat obesity.

Should You Ditch the Dark Chocolates Too?

Dark chocolate at one time was put in the corner shelves, since it was only considered a delicacy for an elite few. However, increasing studies show the health giving benefits of dark chocolate. The fact that most of the health benefits of dark chocolate have been supported by various studies done not only by major chocolate manufacturers, but also independently indicate that there is some truth that dark chocolate is indeed good for health.

There are various health benefits from eating dark chocolate. The key ingredient that makes all the difference in dark chocolate is the high level of cocoa that remains in it after processing. The problem is that most manufacturers remove most of the cocoa during the manufacturing process and replace it with milk solids, sugar, and other additives. The heating process too negates the positive effects of cocoa to a great extent.

Dark chocolate can taste bittersweet, but the positive effects of this cocoa laden delicacy could be sweet music to your ears. One of its miracle properties is the ability to reduce blood pressure. Studies by German doctors among various others have shown that dark chocolate contains cocoa polyphenols, which is responsible for reducing blood pressure without changing one's body weight. Even though the reduction may not be too drastic, eating dark chocolate is one tasty way of reducing blood pressure.

Dark chocolate has also shown to improve the function of the heart by relaxing arteries and also improving their response. The antioxidants present in dark chocolates also prevent free radicals from harming the heart by causing heart diseases. There are various levels of cocoa present in dark chocolate and if possible, you should choose the one with the maximum cocoa content, since it has higher benefits as compared to chocolate with lower levels of cocoa. The downside is that cocoa in its unsweetened form is quite bitter, and hence you will need to balance out between taste and benefits.

Dark chocolate can also reduce the levels of bad cholesterol [LDL]. It can also help in reducing weight, since cocoa is known to reduce appetite and its intake can result in an increase in energy. Dark chocolate also contains fiber, which helps the digestion system to digest food in an efficient manner. Dark chocolate also contains magnesium, which in addition helps to reduce blood pressure, also helps to reduce diabetes, stroke and osteoporosis. The cocoa in dark chocolate can also act as mood enhancers by increasing the brain's dopamine activity. There is however, one fact that should not be ignored before you start munching down dark chocolate.

Dark chocolate contains high calories that can pile on extra flab on to your body. Hence, as in everything else in life, moderation is the key word. Although, dark chocolate does have many health benefits and should definitely be a part of your lifestyle, it is important to remember that a healthy balance is required to balance out the high calories in dark chocolate by eating other healthy foods, in order to maintain a healthy calorie intake. Thus, dark chocolate is indeed a bittersweet miracle that if taken wisely can truly benefit your body and mind.

Does Hypnosis Therapy Help?

People have tried various ways and chalked out diets in their bid to lose weight and eat healthy food. While exercises do help largely, healthy eating habits are equally important, since you will not lose any calories, if you eat four donuts or a slab of chocolate after every workout.

The biggest hurdle to develop healthy eating habits is will power, since many people are not able to hold on to their scheduled diet for a long time. Since will power is just convincing your mind to stick to a particular diet, hypnosis or hypnotherapy is just a method of re-directing or re-programming your mind to veer towards eating healthy food, while reducing the craving for sugar-rich and fried foods. Even as diet programs, diet pills or diet drinks might try to address your problem at a superficial level, hypnosis therapy can root out the problem by eliminating the desire for unhealthy high-fat foods.

Hypnosis therapy tries to reach into the unconscious or subconscious area of the brain, where all these cravings are embedded and tries to either eliminate or re-direct those feelings, towards eating healthy foods. The problem is that your subconscious mind could be accustomed to eating unhealthy foods since childhood and as different people have different reasons for eating unhealthy foods, it is important to recognize the correct reason for the lack of motivation, before it can be treated. If you are not eating healthy food due to any specific reason, such as due to depression or if you see eating high-calorie foods as a reward for any successful action, then your therapist can hypnotize you and find out the actual reason.

Hypnosis therapy can thus directly communicate with your subconscious level of your brain to find the actual reasons for the failure to stick to a particular diet or the reasons behind the addiction to any particular unhealthy food group. Once the therapist configures the real reason for your eating problems, the next step is to reconfigure the brain to hone in on healthy foods and proper eating habits, and even feel content, while eating smaller portions of food.

The results might not be visible instantly, but instead it could be visible over a period of increasing sessions with the therapist. However, it is still better than popping slimming pills or drinks over a period of years without achieving any consistent results. Until you have a long-term motivation to remain healthy, the short-term objectives will only result in a yo-yo effect on your health.

Hypnosis therapy can thus overcome the will power problem and empower your brain towards a new and healthy lifestyle. However, not all people can be successfully hypnotized and your therapist would be in a better position to predict the success ratings for your particular case.

Hypnosis therapy can thus get into the subconscious area of your mind and in addition to removing the craving for unhealthy foods in unhealthy quantities, can also encourage your mind to crave for healthy foods and a healthy lifestyle. Hypnosis therapy can thus eliminate your eating problems from the root and plant a new sapling that encourages you to stick to healthy eating.

How to Start Eating Healthy Today

Is the food you eat healthy? Does it contain all the proteins, minerals and vitamins essentials? If you don't already know, it's high time you realize what exactly you are consuming. The three meals of the day have to be healthy and on time; if possible stretch them to five or six smaller meals. If you are a working in an office or are a salesperson, you will tend to order some fast food, as and when you are hungry. This is a very unhealthy idea.

Make an effort, and cook something healthy. If you don't know how to cook or have any recipes, you can always search online. Many sites give you detailed recipes for vegetarian and non-vegetarian cooking. Salads with fruits and vegetables are a very healthy meal for all ages. It provides you with a lot of energy and keeps you fit. A lot of doctors and dieticians recommend salad meal at least once in a day. If you get bored eating the same salad every day, add new flavors, and bring in a greater variety and try different methods of preparing salads. Grilled, baked, and steamed food is always advisable.

Many people do not eat healthy because most of them cannot give up the foods they like, which is fattening, but tasty. You can always add non-vegetarian items like boiled chicken, grilled pieces of steak, egg white and grilled bacon. This is mainly for people, who do not want to give up on steak and bacon easily. You can always search online for healthy recipes of foods that contain your favorite steak, bacon, ham, etc. Avoid eating fat content foods like egg yolk, bread, rice, sugar and sweets.

Try brown and whole wheat bread and brown rice and brown sugar instead. There is always a healthy alternative for your taste of food. In your recipes, always use ingredients that are sugar free, cholesterol free and fat free. This helps you remain fit and reduces risks to your cardio vascular system.

Know simple facts like:

•Avoid using too much oil

•Do not overeat

•Use right ingredients

•White, and lean meats are better than fatty red meat

•Dairy based products are fattening

•Avoid deep fried foods

•Processed food is not all that great, though it might taste good

•Junk food is filling but not healthy.

•Olive oil is the best cooking medium, if at all you want to deep-fry something.

•Instead of frying, stir-fry your vegetables.

Find time to search for food facts, what alternatives you can have etc. Learn ways to make meals with less fattening and yet healthy and tasty. Remember it's not only for you, but your family as well. Your recipe should never contain a lot of non-vegetarian food, especially if you are serving dinner because non-vegetarian food takes a bit longer to digest. Fruits and vegetables in all your food are healthy. If you have decided to cook and eat healthy food, check the difference in your weight, skin, freshness and concentration just in a few weeks.

CHAPTER 10- HEALTHY EATING PLANS FOR SPECIAL CASES

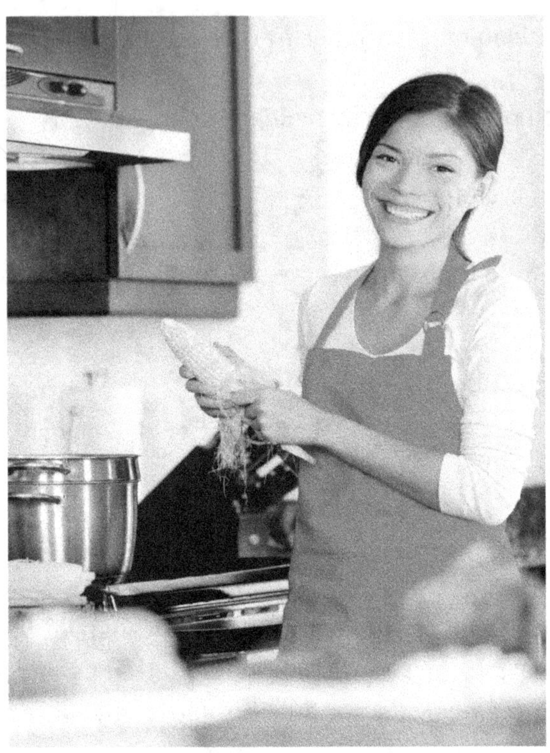

For the Diabetic

A diabetic has to be very careful of the foods consumed, as it is a malfunction, where a body loses its control over producing insulin, and the glucose level in the body fluctuates. A diabetic's diet plan is different from, the normal, because many essential foods contain sugar and these foods need elimination from a diabetic's list.

So, if you are diabetic, refer to a registered dietician or food counsellor.

Diet plan:

Plan your diet. Write down all the food you like and eat. Segregate those with sugar content. With this process, you know what exactly you can consume, and at what rate. Your diet plan must include proper food, and meal timings. Take the help of your doctor or dietician to prepare this plan. Check your blood pressure, blood sugar levels, weight, etc., before you draw your diet plan. From the total calories consumed in a day, an average diabetic should target about 55% of carbohydrates, around 15% of proteins and 30% of fats.

Eating plan:

Your list should include edibles like spinach, bitter gourd, beets etc., as they are supposed to be low in glucose content. Fruits like gooseberry, blackberry, and oranges provide less glucose and more of vitamins. It is advised to eat often, but little and recommended food only. This is because diabetics, when very hungry, can faint. Eat a lot of green leafy vegetables and use fat free food products. Reduce the consumption of alcohol, as it adds sugar to your body. If your sugar level fluctuates, have food that contains adequate amount of carbohydrates.

Here are some tips on how you can manage to reduce the level of sugar content in your body, if you are a diabetic.

• A glass of bitter gourd juice every morning can help you balance your sugar level. If you hate the taste of it, have a glass of orange juice right after that to change the taste of your mouth.

• Eat spinach, and tomatoes with your food.

•A glass of blackberry seed juice is considered a medicine for diabetics in many countries.

•Fenugreek seed juice is again good for diabetics.

If you carefully look, all the above-mentioned food items are bitter in taste or have no sugar content. Consult your doctor or health counsellor before you try any of the above-mentioned tips, as it might differ from person to person. If you have a high level of sugar in your body, completely stop consuming sugar and sweets, and control the level of oil in your food. Many people adhere to junk, oily, spicy and fattening food, while in the process of controlling their sugar levels. They reduce the level of sugar but end up with heart problems. Therefore, it is very necessary to keep a check on your weight and blood pressure along with your sugar level. Eat healthy and reduce the risk, if not eliminate diabetes from your body.

The Elderly

Generally, people in over sixty have altered food tastes. Foods do not taste the same. They lose appetite and even their favorite foods do not fascinate them anymore. They tend to put on weight even if they barely eat. Metabolism rates decrease with age and people tend to put on fats. Increasing weight in sixties is a bad sign, as it can cause many health related hazards. A person in his/her sixties must follow a proper diet plan.

Here are some tips on how you can maintain your weight and diet accordingly.

People usually do not work very hard in their sixties and therefore need less energy, but just enough to perform daily chores. Your diet must contain adequate amount of protein, calcium, carbohydrates and vitamins. Eat different varieties of food every day, so that it does not get monotonous and you have different taste every day.

As you grow old, your bones tend to become weak and feeble. Your calcium level decreases and you are likely to suffer from osteoporosis. To avoid these sufferings, you should drink enough low-fat milk and eat fat free dairy products like cheese and butter.

Make sure you do not gain fat. Fruits and vegetables are a very important source of nutrition for persons of this age group, as they provide a sufficient amount of vitamins and minerals. Most fruits contain vitamins B and C. Vitamins and calcium prevent memory loss, and shivering.

Protein in your diet must only be about 15-18%, and mostly got from non-vegetarian foods like fish, eggs, and meat. Always keep your body hydrated with water and juices. Water helps in cleansing the body from its impurities. Eat fiber rich food like vegetables that provide proteins, too. More of fiber in the body means less of toxins. Fiber can be found in pulses and baked beans, prunes and apricots.

Do not eat a lot of sweet or sugar based food because the empty calories present in them do not exactly provide energy, but increases weight. Consumption of excess salt may raise high blood pressure, therefore, control intakes of salt and sugar.

Since senior people do not exactly engage themselves in physical activity, regular exercise and a proper diet is a must. One has to increase metabolism rate, in order to remain fit and not put on excess weight.

Old people often eat very less and cannot have three big meals. They must have small meals after regular intervals, which helps to increase their metabolism rate. Do not take any protein supplements or fats loss pills because they need vigorous workouts and are basically meant for people below 60.

Avoid canned or packed food items, as they contain preservatives, which are not healthy for persons of that age group. Some packaged food also contains hydrogenated fats that may cause a problem in your cardio-vascular system.

Eat controlled amounts of food, but ensure they are nutrient rich, so that you live a long, healthy life.

The Underweight

A lot is written about weight loss and a slimmer body. However, some are underweight, and constantly look for ways to gain weight. To stay healthy, one needs the perfect weight. Being underweight is equally bad for your body. If you have tried to gain weight and failed every attempt, the reason may be that either you are following a wrong path or you are just not following the method. Your body weight depends on what you eat.

Eating unhealthy stuff can lead to weight loss and make you look pale and sick. When the body is deprived of proper meals, it will start eating the cells within the body making you lose your body mass. Do you know that every time your body makes any movements, it loses calories? There are many people, who have a busy and hectic life, but simply fail to eat and neglect to eat what the body requires. Eating healthy meals and at proper time will help you gain the perfect body shape that you have been wishing for.

If you fall in the category of underweight persons, firstly, alter your diet and include foods that are more nutritious. Have small meals, but take it at least 4 to 5 times a day. Apart from altering your diet, you need to change your eating habits as well. You can't keep eating as you wish. You should understand your body clock and work accordingly. Long gaps between meals are as good as starving, and destroy your cells. Plan out a schedule to eat and follow it accordingly. Frequent changes affect the body adversely and make you lose more energy and body mass. Begin your day with a glass of milk and cereals, and then eat fruits. Prepare a few vegetable sandwiches with butter or cheese.

Remember to take your breakfast, soon after you wake up. There should also be less time gap between your breakfast and lunch. If for any reason it takes time, grab a fruit or a healthy drink or a nutritious bar to munch. It is good to make salads as part of your meals. A large portion of chicken or fish is healthy and helps you gain weight as well. It is a good idea to include some green leafy vegetables in your meals. Do take a snack break in the evening and pamper yourself with some protein drink and healthy sandwiches or salad.

If at any time you happen to do some heavy activities, remember your body has burnt lots of calories and thus you need to recharge by eating something healthy. Include a lot of liquids in your diet as well, so that the body keeps getting the required amount of liquid to flush out the unwanted toxins and keep your stomach clean. Combining healthy eating with exercise will do wonders for your body.

A good diet will not only help you gain weight, but also make you look great. When your energy levels are high, you feel fresh throughout the day and can undertake any task with ease. A healthy body and mind can do lots of good. Eat right and stay fit and you will enjoy life like never before. If you have a balanced diet, you need not consume weight gain powders or tablets. A proper diet should work perfectly on your body. Nothing is as great as eating good, wholesome food.

The Infants

As a parent, you must take a number of precautions about your infant's diet. The best food for an infant is mother's milk. Normally, an infant is considered as baby of age 0 – 1 year old. People even consider preschoolers as infants.

Let us categorize infants in different age groups and discuss their diet and precautions taken.

0-4 months:

From the day of birth until the infant is 4 months, there is no better food for the child than the mother's milk. Mother's milk contains all the essentials that a child needs in balanced amounts. The temperature, thinness of milk, germ fighting and immunity enhancers, and many other factors ideal for the infant are present in mother's milk. At this time, an infant is not ready to digest solid or semi-solid foods; therefore, continue breast-feeding until 4-5 months. Even if the baby gets diarrhea, continue breast-feeding. It is best to continue breast-feeding the child up to the age of one year, but in this age, it is not possible.

5-6 months:

You can now introduce your child to semi-solid food. At this age, the baby is not completely ready to ingest semi-solid food, but is partially all right. Try to feed the baby with cereals like wheat, maize or mashed fruits like apples. Make sure you dilute the food with either mother's milk or water. Feed the infant porridges. Feed the infant small amounts to a time, until it no longer is hungry.

Do not force feed your infant, as it might initially not eat and might throw up. This happens because the infant is used only to sucking. The infant's food intake will gradually increase. Do not stop breast-feeding. When your infant opens his/her mouth while feeding or the eyes follow the spoon means, your baby is now ready to taste and eat new food. Always feed your baby on your lap, this gives them the feeling of security.

7-9 months:

After the baby gives positive response to the semi-solid food, you can now bring in mild solid food. Extremely small and fine pieces of fruits and vegetables, soft cheese, thin pieces of chicken should be the child's meal. Initially the child might not be very happy biting the food and might not eat. Therefore it is advised not to stop breast-feeding. If your baby is hungry every 2-4 hours and wets the diapers 4-6 times a day, it means, your baby is getting food and fluids in right quantity. Other indication could be baby's weight increase.

10-12 months: The food in this period is not so different, but a little variation in the food is required. Bigger chopped piece of meat, fish, vegetables and fruits could be given. Cereals, mother's milk and fruit juices diluted with water are recommended as liquids. Always introduce new foods after every 2 weeks. This helps you spot the food types that cause allergies or illness to your child. Maintain a high level of hygiene. Always boil water; always feed lukewarm food.

ABOUT THE AUTHOR

Kevin Jones is a nutritionist and a chef. He owns and runs his own restaurant, where he serves fresh meals with their nutritional values in mind.

This is Kevin's first published work but he hopes to write many more.

Kevin has a daughter, Patty.